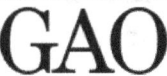

I0415885

June 2012

PATIENT PROTECTION AND AFFORDABLE CARE ACT

IRS Managing Implementation Risks, but Its Approach Could Be Refined

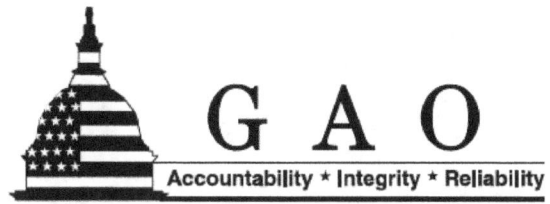

GAO

Accountability * Integrity * Reliability

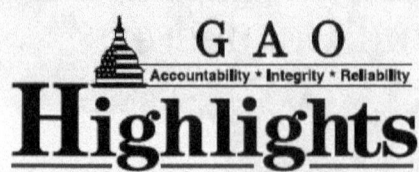
June 2012

PATIENT PROTECTION AND AFFORDABLE CARE ACT

IRS Managing Implementation Risks, but Its Approach Could Be Refined

Why GAO Did This Study

PPACA is a significant effort for IRS, with expected costs of $881 million from fiscal years 2010 to 2013 and work planned through 2018. To implement PPACA, IRS must work closely with partner agencies to develop information technology systems that can share data with other agencies. Additionally, IRS is responsible for providing guidance to taxpayers, employers, insurers, and others to ensure compliance with new tax aspects of the law. Furthermore, it will be important for IRS to have systems to consistently identify, assess, mitigate, and monitor potential risks to the program's success.

As requested, this report (1) describes IRS's progress in addressing GAO recommendations from June 2011 on PPACA implementation, (2) assesses IRS's revised risk management plan, and (3) assesses how IRS applies its plan in practice. GAO compared IRS's revised risk plan to GAO's criteria for risk management and selected 9 provisions of the law in which IRS had a role to determine whether IRS used the risk plan consistently. Because selection focused on provisions that had the most risks and highest dollar impacts, the results are not generalizable but are relevant to how IRS managed risks.

What GAO Recommends

GAO recommends that IRS (1) enhance its guidance on evaluating risk mitigation alternatives and documenting decisions, (2) use a risk management plan for work led by its Office of Chief Counsel, and (3) develop agreements with external parties to record and track risks that threaten shared goals and objectives. IRS officials agreed with all of GAO's recommendations.

View GAO-12-690. For more information, contact James R. White at (202) 512-9110 or whitej@gao.gov.

What GAO Found

The Internal Revenue Service (IRS) has implemented one of GAO's four recommendations from June 2011 to strengthen the Patient Protection and Affordable Care Act (PPACA) implementation efforts by scheduling the development of performance measures for the PPACA program. IRS has made varying degrees of progress on the other three recommendations:

- develop program goals and an integrated project plan;
- develop a cost estimate consistent with GAO's published guidance; and
- assure that IRS's risk management plan identifies strategic level risks and evaluates associated mitigation options.

IRS's revised risk management plan meets three of five criteria for risk management plans, but the plan does not have specific guidance for evaluating and selecting potential risk mitigation options, such as how to

- identify who conducts and reviews the analysis,
- determine the availability of resources for a given strategy, and
- document for future users the rationale behind decisions made.

IRS applied its risk management plan when identifying, tracking, and reporting on implementation risks. Although the risk plan calls for risk mitigation strategies to be evaluated, these evaluations have not been done. IRS officials said that evaluating these strategies would require varying levels of effort because the probability and magnitude of risks differ. However, the plan was silent on this point; it provided no guidance as to when and to what extent an evaluation should be done. Without evaluating potential strategies, IRS may not consider critical factors that impact the program's success.

IRS's risk management plan was not used when IRS's Office of Chief Counsel was responsible for implementing two provisions GAO reviewed. Although these provisions primarily required legal counsel and guidance, IRS officials said that one of the provisions also affected IRS operations and could have risks that need to be managed. Additionally, GAO did not find evidence that a risk plan was used to track and mitigate risks when coordinating with partner agencies, such as the Department of Health and Human Services. Without a system for tracking shared risks, IRS is more likely to overlook risks or duplicate efforts.

Contents

Figures

Abbreviations

AGI	Adjusted Gross Income
BOD	Business Operating Division
CFO	Office of the Chief Financial Officer
EPO	Estimating Program Office
ESC	Executive Steering Committee
FTE	full-time equivalent
HCERA	Health Care and Education Reconciliation Act of 2010
HHS	Department of Health and Human Services
HIRIF	Health Insurance Reform Implementation Fund
HLAP	high level action plan
IRS	Internal Revenue Service
IT	information technology
LB&I	Large Business & International Division
MITS	Modernization and Information Technology Services
PMO	Program Management Office
PPACA	Patient Protection and Affordable Care Act
RAS	Research Analysis and Statistics
S&E	Services and Enforcement
SB/SE	Small Business/Self-Employed Division
TE/GE	Tax Exempt/Government Entities Division
W&I	Wages & Investment Division

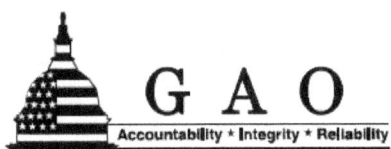

United States Government Accountability Office
Washington, DC 20548

June 13, 2012

The Honorable Richard J. Durbin
Chairman
The Honorable Jerry Moran
Ranking Member
Subcommittee on Financial Services and General Government
Committee on Appropriations
United States Senate

The Honorable Sam Graves
Chairman
Committee on Small Business
House of Representatives

The Internal Revenue Service's (IRS) implementation of the Patient Protection and Affordable Care Act (PPACA)[1] is a massive undertaking that involves 47 statutory provisions and extensive coordination across not only IRS, but multiple agencies and external partners. For example, IRS must coordinate with other federal agencies and states in providing assistance to qualifying individuals for health insurance premiums. In June 2011, we reported that IRS had generally followed leading practices for implementing such a large program, particularly at the level of individual offices and projects, and we made four recommendations to improve IRS's strategic approach to its implementation efforts.[2]

IRS has continued to make progress implementing PPACA. However, a number of risks remain. In particular, IRS must quickly design and implement large information technology (IT) systems used to carry out key provisions of the law. The investment is large, as IRS's implementation costs from fiscal years 2010 through 2013 are expected to total $881 million. IRS also plays a critical role in helping individuals, employers, insurers, health care providers, tax practitioners, state agencies, and other federal agencies understand their obligations under

---

[1] Pub. L. No. 111-148, 124 Stat. 119 (March 23, 2010) as amended by the Health Care and Education Reconciliation Act of 2010 (Pub. L. No. 111-152).

[2] GAO, *Patient Protection and Affordable Care Act: IRS Should Expand Its Strategic Approach to Implementation*, GAO-11-719 (Washington, D.C.: June 25, 2011).

the law and in ensuring compliance while minimizing the burden of complying.

As we emphasized in our June 2011 report, effective management of these efforts requires significant long-term planning by IRS to ensure a comprehensive system for managing and mitigating risks and monitoring progress. Doing so requires IRS to coordinate efforts internally as well as with outside partners, such as the Department of Health and Human Services (HHS), so that all parties understand what they need to do and when to do it (accounting for changes necessary) in a manner that keeps the overall implementation on track. Efforts to manage risk over the long-term led IRS to create a risk management plan specifically for the PPACA program, which IRS revised most recently in February of 2012.

Given your interests in tracking IRS's progress in implementing its responsibilities while managing various risks, you asked us to review IRS's progress since our June 2011 report and assess IRS's risk management. In this report we (1) describe IRS's progress in acting on our four recommendations, (2) assess IRS's use of leading practices in its revised risk management plan,[3] and (3) assess how IRS follows its risk management plan for a sample of PPACA provisions as well as for four crosscutting management areas: allocating resources, coordinating with partner agencies, determining the need for deadline extensions, and assuring compliance with the law while minimizing burden.

To assess IRS's progress in implementing our recommendations, we met with responsible IRS executives and staff and reviewed IRS documentation, comparing IRS's planned and ongoing actions to the leading practices discussed in our 2011 report. To assess how IRS designed its plan, we compared IRS's actions to guidelines set by GAO's risk management approach. We interviewed IRS management and staff about these guidelines and collected documentation on IRS's adherence. To assess how IRS manages risks for the four key areas, we compared IRS actions to the guidelines outlined in its risk management plan. As part of this work, we analyzed how IRS adhered to these guidelines in implementing 9 provisions that we selected from the IRS-related

---

[3] For purposes of this report, we used leading practices from GAO's risk management approach to assess IRS's risk management plan. See GAO, *Risk Management: Further Refinements Needed to Assess Risks and Prioritize Protective Measures at Ports and Other Critical Infrastructure,* GAO-06-91 (Washington, D.C.: Dec. 15, 2005).

provisions that involved the highest dollar amounts.[4] For details on our methodology, including the selection of the provisions in our sample, see appendix I.

We conducted this performance audit from August 2011 through June 2012 in accordance with generally accepted government auditing standards. These standards require that we plan and perform the audit to obtain sufficient, appropriate evidence to provide a reasonable basis for our findings and conclusions based on our audit objectives. We believe that the evidence obtained provides a reasonable basis for our findings and conclusions based on our audit objectives.

Background

Enacted on March 23, 2010, PPACA involves major health care stakeholders, including federal and state governments, employers, insurers, and health care providers, in an attempt to reform the private insurance market and expand health coverage to the uninsured. IRS is one of several agencies accountable for implementing the legislation and has responsibilities pertaining to 47 PPACA provisions.[5] Some provisions took effect immediately or retroactively while others are to take effect as late as 2018.

According to IRS officials, the most challenging of these provisions relate to the health care exchanges to be established by states by 2014. These exchanges are marketplaces for individuals and certain types of employers to purchase health insurance. To support the exchanges, IRS must modify existing or design new IT systems that are capable of transmitting data to and from HHS, help HHS craft eligibility determinations and related definitions, and engage in new interagency coordination, such as with HHS and the Department of Labor.

---

[4] Applying these criteria separately to the 47 provisions, 23 provisions were scored to have revenue or spending impacts of over $1 billion by the Joint Committee on Taxation and Congressional Budget Office. We identified provisions that were implemented when the risk plan was in place and that had multiple, significant risks to narrow this pool of provisions to a judgmental sample of 9.

[5] This number does not include a provision from section 9006 of the law calling for expanded information reporting to payments made to corporations and to payments for property and other gross proceeds. The requirements of this provision were repealed on April 14, 2011 by the Comprehensive 1099 Taxpayer Protection and Repayment of Exchange Subsidy Overpayments Act of 2011, Pub. L. No. 112-9.

To coordinate agency-wide efforts, a PPACA Executive Steering Committee (ESC) oversees two Program Management Offices (PMOs) that coordinate with Health Care Counsel—which is part of IRS's Office of Chief Counsel (Counsel)[6]—on the implementation.[7] The Services and Enforcement (S&E) PMO oversees the work completed within IRS's existing business operating divisions (BOD)[8] as well as the efforts of four workstream teams. The Modernization, Information Technology and Security Services (MITS) PMO leads IT development for the program. The Health Care Counsel provides legal counsel and guidance (see fig. 1). Management of the implementation teams is expected to shift from the program management office to the business operating divisions, MITS, and Counsel as the program is fully implemented.

---

[6] The IRS Chief Counsel also reports to the United States Department of the Treasury General Counsel on certain matters.

[7] See GAO-11-719.

[8] BODs include: Wage & Investment Division (W&I), Small Business/Self-Employed Division (SB/SE), Large Business & International Division (LB&I), and Tax Exempt/Government Entities Division (TE/GE).

GAO-12-690 Patient Protection and Affordable Care Act

Figure 1: IRS PPACA Organization Chart

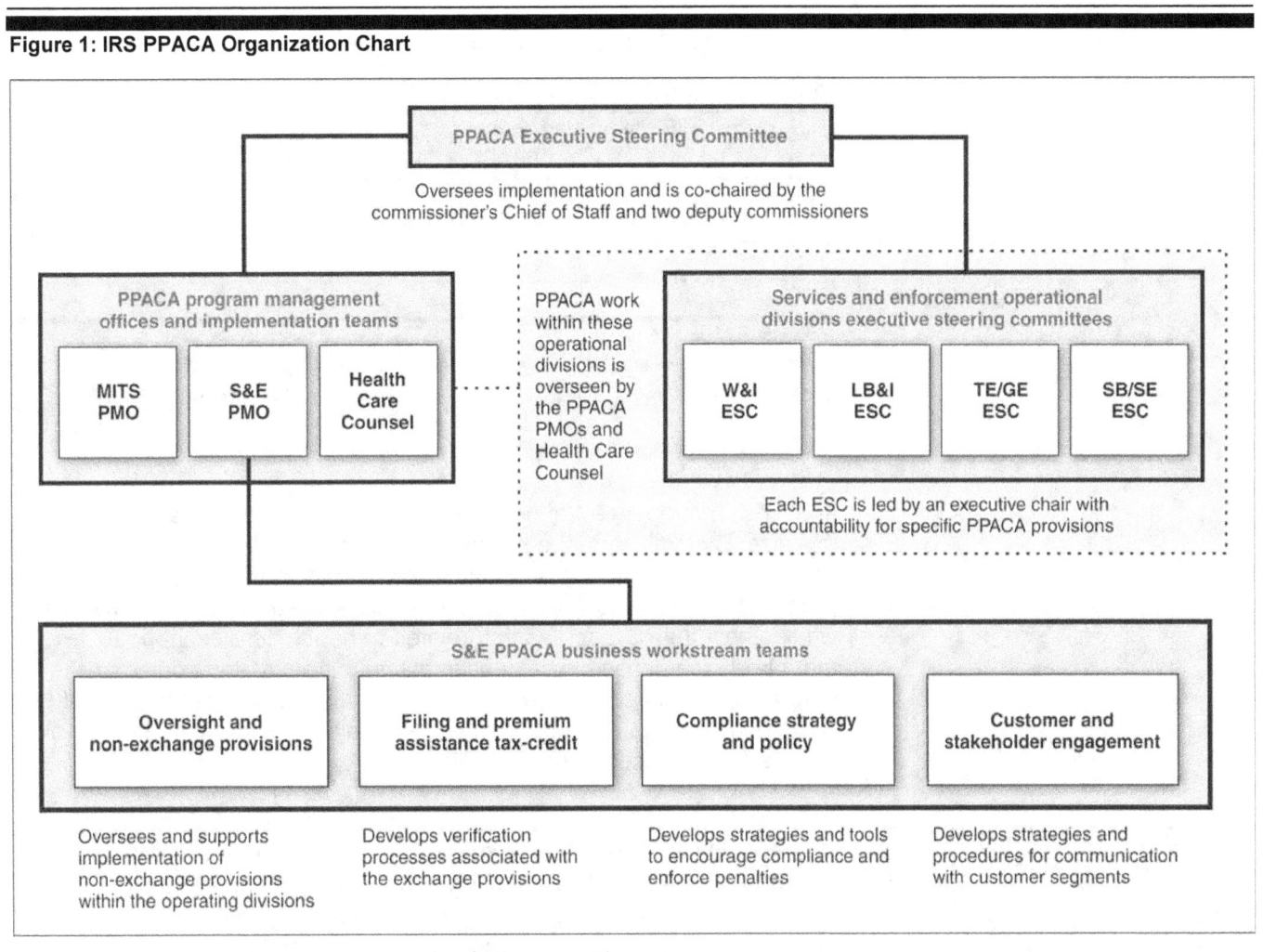

Source: GAO analysis of IRS documentation.

The program management offices and business operating divisions, along with overall IRS leadership, coordinate with IRS's Office of the Chief Financial Officer (CFO) to allocate resources for implementation efforts. Implementation costs are expected to reach $881 million through fiscal year 2013, with $521 million of that amount being provided through HHS's Health Insurance Reform Implementation Fund (HIRIF), a fund to which Congress appropriated $1 billion for federal spending to implement PPACA, and the remainder from IRS's 2013 budget request. Table 1 shows IRS's PPACA budget and HIRIF funding amounts.

Table 1: IRS PPACA Budget and HIRIF Funding, Fiscal Years 2010 to 2013

Dollars in millions

Fiscal year	IRS requested budget for PPACA	IRS enacted budget for PPACA	HIRIF funding
2010	a	$0	$21
2011	a	$0	$168
2012	$473	$0	$332[b]
2013	$360	c	c

Source: IRS.

[a]PPACA was enacted after IRS requested funding for fiscal years 2010 and 2011.

[b]IRS requested $332 million from the HIRIF for fiscal year 2012 and had received $135 million as of April 27, 2012.

[c]The figures were undetermined at the time of our report.

IRS's risk management efforts are crucial in implementing a program of this size. By evaluating the probability and impact of a given risk's occurrence, risk management encourages planning for ways to lessen the probability or minimize the impact. Much of the remaining implementation work is new to IRS, such as that related to health care exchanges. IRS is more likely to succeed with steps in place to identify and address risks before they occur and make contingency plans for events that cannot be controlled. Though not a guarantee, IRS's planning for these tasks make successful implementation more likely.

IRS Has Made Varying Degrees of Progress in Implementing Our Recommendations but Has More to Do on Project Planning, Cost Estimating, and Evaluating Risk Mitigation Strategies

Over half of the 47 provisions requiring action from IRS were statutorily effective in or prior to 2010, forcing IRS to conduct short-term implementations and long-term strategic planning simultaneously. With many short-term projects now completed, IRS has been focusing on its long-term planning since our 2011 report, and has made varying degrees of progress in implementing our four recommendations. These efforts have helped IRS gain a better understanding and vision for the implementation work and challenges remaining and how IRS would manage risks to the program's success.

IRS has implemented one of our four recommendations from June 2011 to strengthen PPACA implementation efforts by documenting a schedule for developing performance measures for PPACA that are to link to program goals (see table 2).

Table 2: Recommendation Status: Developing a Plan to Create Performance Measures

Criteria for meeting recommendation	IRS status in 2012
1. Articulate the actions required in developing performance measures. Steps to be taken should be documented so that progress can be tracked.	Met: Planning document lists actions to take in developing performance measures.
2. Establish dates by which actions will be completed. Deadline dates should be specific.	Met: Deadline is July 1, 2012.

Source: GAO analysis based on GAO reports and IRS documentation.

IRS made some progress on the remaining three recommendations from our June 2011 report. Absent more progress, IRS may encounter challenges in overseeing the program if activities in project plans are not linked, cost estimates are not current, and risk mitigation strategies are not properly assessed and decisions documented.

Integrating Goals and Project Plan

We recommended that IRS develop one set of goals and an integrated project plan across IRS to clarify the vision and mitigate the risk that lower level units may work at cross purposes. The program's governance document now stipulates program goals that align with IRS's mission. IRS continues to maintain separate project plans for S&E and MITS activities, though it has an additional plan that offers a high level overview of the major PPACA efforts and the related implementation progress across IRS. IRS officials said that the overview provides a sufficient perspective to assess overall progress, but we found it did not align with criteria for leading practices because it is updated manually, leaving it subject to error if those updating the plan are not acting in a timely manner or overlook a change in delivery schedules (see table 3).

GAO-12-690 Patient Protection and Affordable Care Act

Table 3: Recommendation Status: Integrating Goals and Project Plans

Criteria for meeting recommendation	IRS status in 2012
1. Goals should link to the agency mission. Program goals should be documented and show a clear link to the agency's mission.	Met: Goals and objectives in Governance Plan link to IRS's mission.
2. Goals should communicate a clear vision of the desired outcome. Documentation should show how expectations for desired program outcomes are communicated.	Met: Governance Plan includes PPACA vision and guiding principles in implementation.
3. Goals should be established by key stakeholders managing the program and approved by the main leadership body for the program.	Met: Governance Plan created by PPACA ESC.
4. Responsibilities and completion dates should be clearly described and documented; the schedule should realistically reflect what resources are needed to do the work and determine whether all required resources will be available when needed.	Partially met: High level plan has appropriate detail of responsibilities and completion dates; relatively few activities have been assigned specific resources.
5. The project plan should articulate a clear system of coordination among project activities. Project schedules should link to recognize impacts of delays and major handoffs and deliverables should be easily identified.	Partially met: Major milestones and deliverables are clear; activities and milestones are not linked electronically; project schedules between S&E and MITS are not linked electronically.
6. The project plan should track results. Schedule progress should be reported periodically and updated regularly. The schedule history should be maintained with narrative for any delays, changes, additions, or deletions of activities. The schedule should compare a baseline plan to current status.	Partially met: Progress is reported periodically; history of actual completion dates is not maintained; no evidence of written narratives for changes to plan; MITS compares current status to a baseline plan, but S&E does not.

Source: GAO analysis based on GAO reports and IRS documentation.

Developing a More Complete Cost Estimate

We recommended that IRS adopt the leading practices outlined in the GAO *Cost Guide*[9] and shown in table 4 to enhance the reliability of its cost estimate for PPACA. However, little progress has been made as IRS's cost estimate is largely unchanged since it was developed in 2010. IRS's Estimating Program Office (EPO) plans to revise the cost estimate this year after reaching a milestone that clarified some business requirements related to IT development. In April 2012, IRS awarded a contract for an independent cost estimate that is slated to include the steps outlined in GAO's *Cost Guide*. Our June 2012 report on IRS's fiscal year 2013 budget recommended that IRS revise its PPACA cost estimate by September 2012, which IRS agreed to do.[10] If IRS's EPO completes

[9] GAO, *Cost Estimating and Assessment Guide: Best Practices for Developing and Managing Capital Program Costs*, GAO-09-3SP (Washington, D.C.: March 2009).

[10] GAO, *IRS 2013 Budget: Continuing to Improve Information on Program Costs and Results Could Aid in Resource Decision Making*, GAO-12-603 (Washington, D.C.: June 8, 2012).

an estimate and it is compared to an independent estimate, IRS will make significant progress in implementing our recommendation.

Table 4: Recommendation Status: Developing a More Complete Cost Estimate

Criteria for meeting recommendation	IRS status in 2012
1. Estimates should be comprehensive: including all life cycle costs and a logical work breakdown structure; completely defining the program; and detailing all ground rules and assumptions.	Partially met: Documents ground rules and assumptions, but not the entire life cycle; Detail of the work necessary does not capture all costs.
2. Estimates should be well-documented: identifying data sources and data reliability; describing all estimating methods; showing step-by-step cost calculations; documenting review and approval from management; and discussing how the technical description is incorporated in the estimate.	Partially met: Methodologies behind calculations are described, though several sources of data are unclear or rely on IRS employee input. Historical data are not normalized to ensure consistency of cost data.
3. Estimates should be accurate: unbiased and based on most likely and historical costs; adjusted for inflation; free from errors; updated regularly; and capable of being analyzed for variance between planned and actual costs.	Partially met: Estimate is unbiased and based on most likely and historical costs, though it was last updated in October 2010. Analysis of variance between actual and projected costs is not documented.
4. Estimates should be credible: including sensitivity, risk, and uncertainty analysis; using more than one method in calculating major cost elements to see if results are similar; and comparing results to independent cost estimate.	Minimally met: IRS statement of work for a cost estimate includes risk and sensitivity analysis, which would help identify variables most likely to affect the estimate. IRS plans to obtain an independent cost estimate in 2012.

Source: GAO analysis based on GAO reports and IRS documentation.

Enhancing Risk Management Plan

We recommended that IRS's plan assure that strategic-level risks are identified and that alternative mitigation strategies for risks are evaluated. Our conclusion was based on a comparison between IRS's risk plan from May 18, 2011, and the criteria outlined in GAO's risk management framework, shown in figure 2.

Figure 2: Risk Management Framework Stages

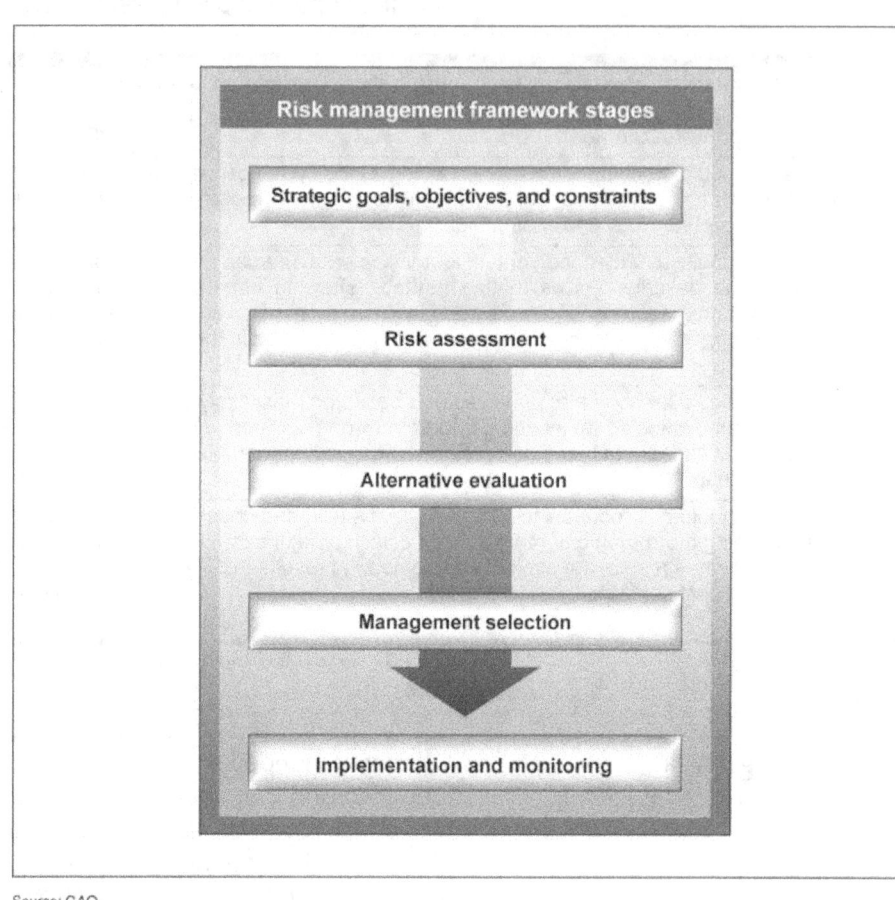

Source: GAO.

Of the five stages of the risk management framework, IRS's risk plan did not meet the criteria associated with three stages: risk assessment, alternative evaluation, and management selection (see table 5). Strategic-level risks are now better addressed because the revised plan calls for involvement of higher level executives, but the plan does not specify policies and procedures involved in evaluating and selecting potential risk mitigation strategies. We discuss this topic further in the next section on IRS's revised risk management plan.

Table 5: Recommendations and IRS Status in 2012 for Enhancing IRS's Managing of Risk

Criteria for meeting recommendation	IRS status in 2012
1. Involve high-level management in identifying program risks. The plan should not rely solely on project teams to identify risks, as cross-cutting risks may be overlooked.	Met: Risk plan states that all PPACA members, including executives, can identify risks.
2. Include procedures for identifying and evaluating mitigation strategies in the plan. Cost-benefit analysis of mitigation options should be done.	Partially met: Risk plan calls for selecting a mitigation approach after identifying alternatives and considering such factors as cost, effort, and return on investment. However, the plan does not provide guidance for performing the analysis, such as who does it and who reviews it.
3. Include procedures for selecting mitigation strategies in the plan and documenting the rationale for decisions made.	Not met: Risk plan does not provide guidance for selecting strategies or call for documenting decisions and the related rationale.

Source: GAO analysis based on GAO reports and IRS documentation.

IRS's Risk Management Plan Meets Criteria for Three of Five Risk Framework Stages but Lacks Specific Guidance on the Evaluation and Selection of Mitigation Strategies

Our assessment of IRS's revised risk management plan from February 24, 2012, indicated that IRS adheres to the criteria for three of the five stages of our framework for risk management. However, the plan's guidance on evaluating risk mitigation alternatives is not specific or comprehensive, nor does the plan address procedures for management in selecting strategies and documenting decisions made. Figure 3 summarizes our assessment of the IRS revised plan by comparing it to the five stages (see app. II for the full text included in fig. 3).

Figure 3: How IRS Fulfills GAO Risk Management Criteria

Directions:

👆 Roll over risk management framework stages below to see how IRS fulfills GAO criteria.

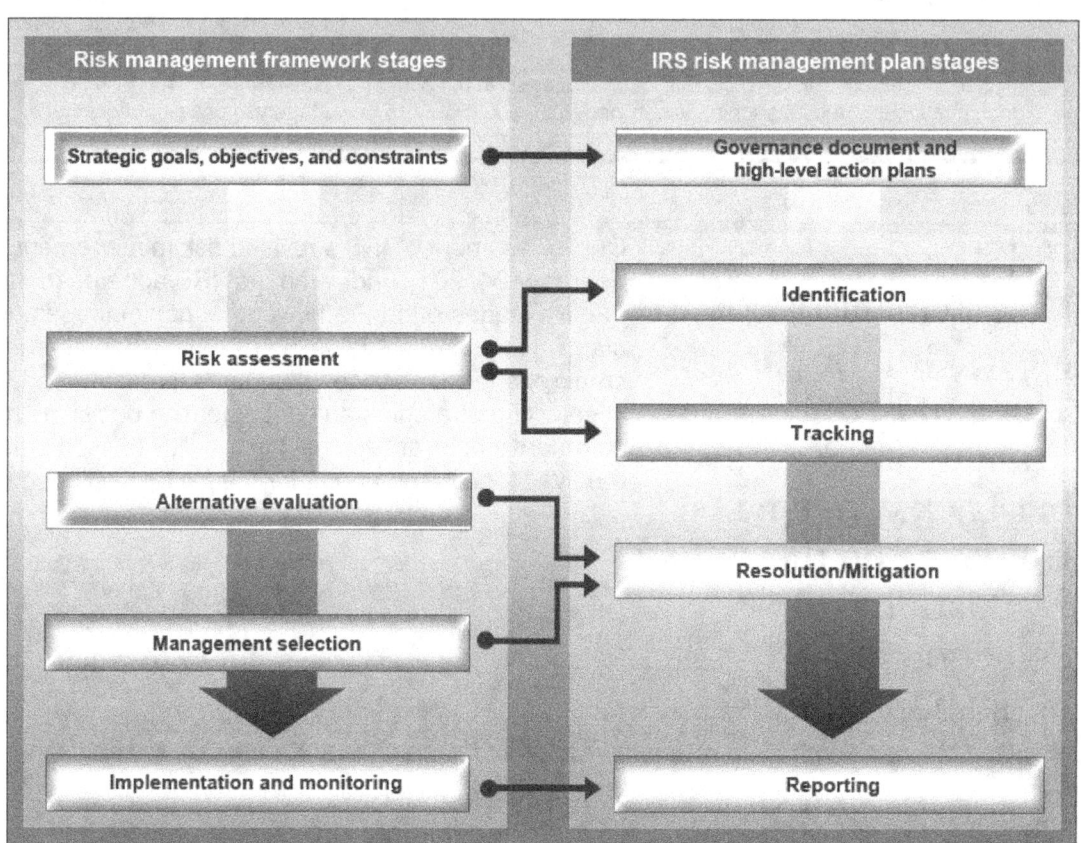

Source: GAO analysis of IRS documentation.

As figure 3 indicates, the risk plan's discussion of evaluating potential risk mitigations is brief, with some processes and responsibilities left undefined. The plan did not provide specific guidance on the process for doing an evaluation, stating only that alternative strategies should be evaluated according to cost, level of effort, and return on investment. For example, the plan did not identify who is responsible for doing or reviewing the evaluation.

Further, the plan did not provide guidance on selecting mitigation strategies, including verifying that resources are available for selected strategies. IRS officials acknowledged that the plan did not include these processes and responsibilities but said that they believe that teams considered such factors when making decisions. Additionally, the plan did not provide guidance on documenting the rationale(s) for selecting one alternative over others. As a result, IRS is less likely to have a trail of analysis that explains the decisions to those who work on PPACA projects in the future. Such a trail is important, as PPACA implementation involves many people managing many tasks over a number of years and across multiple offices. In the years ahead, implementation responsibility will shift from the PMOs to staff in the BODs who may not have been involved in these decisions about the mitigations considered and chosen and may have to develop a new mitigation if the original does not work.

IRS officials noted that spending resources to do a thorough evaluation and to document the rationale for decisions may not be practical for risks that have a low probability of occurring or that IRS cannot control, such as a lack of funding. While this may be true, IRS's risk plan does not offer guidance on factors like the probability of a risk's occurrence that could affect the level of evaluation and amount of documentation to be done. Without specific guidance on evaluating potential mitigation strategies, the likelihood decreases that teams will conduct a thorough evaluation or have a consistent basis for deciding not to do so.

IRS Implemented Its Risk Management Plan Consistently for the Sample Provisions and in Crosscutting Areas, Except for Provisions Led by Counsel and When Coordinating with Partner Agencies

Managing Risks for Sample Provisions

Our analysis indicated that IRS generally implemented its risk management plan consistently for seven of the nine provisions in our sample. These seven provisions covered responsibilities such as for premium assistance tax credits for eligible individuals purchasing health insurance coverage through state exchanges, penalties on individuals who do not have minimum essential coverage, penalties on larger employers who do not offer coverage as required, and other taxes, credits, and fees. IRS did not follow its risk management plan for two sample provisions that IRS believed primarily required legal guidance and that IRS assigned primary responsibility for implementing to Counsel.[11]

In reviewing the seven sample provisions that were expected to have relatively high dollar impacts and greater risks, we asked for evidence that IRS completed the steps prescribed by its risk plan.[12] Table 6 summarizes the steps and results we found in IRS's implementation of the plan for the seven provisions (see app. III for detail on the sample provisions and our assessment of whether the sample provisions followed the four stages of IRS's risk plan).

---

[11] Provisions included section 1102 on establishing a temporary reinsurance program for early retirees and section 1409 on the application of the economic substance doctrine. See app. III for a description of these provisions.

[12] Our analyses focused on whether rather than how well IRS completed the required steps.

Table 6: Assessment of IRS's Implementation of Its Risk Plan for Sampled Provisions

Stage of risk plan	Key steps included in the stage	Results found in implementation
Identification	Brainstorming sessions with relevant stakeholders; guidance from Counsel; complete and document approval of Provision Assessment Form; record identified risks in tracking software, using information from Provision Assessment Form.	IRS provided evidence of taking these steps.
Tracking	Monitor risks weekly.	IRS provided evidence of a weekly review meeting for risks.
Resolution/ Mitigation	Determine risk levels for each recorded risk; evaluate and select risk mitigation strategies; assign risk ownership; establish performance thresholds that offer early warning that chosen mitigation strategies do not work.	Risk levels were determined; risk ownership was assigned; little evidence of mitigation strategy evaluation; provisions with earlier effective dates were more likely to have established early warning indicators.
Reporting	Regularly scheduled reports reviewed at meetings by IRS management committees.	IRS provided evidence of taking these steps.

Source: GAO analysis of IRS documentation.

IRS consistently completed all steps outlined in the plan's Identification, Tracking, and Reporting stages. While some steps called for in the Resolution/Mitigation stage were consistently completed, we did not find an analysis of alternative risk mitigation strategies for several provisions in our sample. This inconsistency could stem from the lack of guidance, as previously discussed, on how to do mitigation evaluations, including documenting why a mitigation strategy is selected over the alternatives considered.

As for the two sample provisions that Counsel was responsible for implementing, the risk management plan was not used. When asked about efforts to identify risks for one of the provisions, a Counsel official said that this responsibility rested with the BODs who ultimately would implement the provision. However, the S&E PMO overseeing the work in the BODs told us that Counsel was responsible for the provision's implementation, including managing the related risks. As a result of confusion as to who should take the lead in identifying and mitigating risks for provisions in which Counsel had lead responsibility, risks may not be identified and mitigated. IRS officials acknowledged that the risk plan was not used for these provisions, noting that the provisions were not expected to have an impact on IRS operations. However, one of the two provisions, an imposition of penalties for underpayments attributable to transactions lacking economic substance, had an operational impact in areas such as tax forms, customer service, and compliance checks, indicating that the risk plan should have been used.

Managing Risks for Four Crosscutting Management Areas

Looking more broadly beyond the provisions in our sample, we found that IRS generally implemented its risk management plan in four crosscutting areas: (1) resource allocation, (2) collaboration with other agencies, (3) decisions to extend deadlines or provide transitional relief, and (4) challenges related to addressing compliance and burden. However, IRS did not have a formal system for managing risks when coordinating with HHS.

Managing Risk in Allocating Resources

While we noted in Table 3 that most activities in project plans were not assigned specific resources, IRS's risk plan does facilitate knowledge sharing among the entities involved in allocating resources to the program, with the exception previously stated that it does not provide guidance on verifying that resources are available for selected mitigation strategies. The CFO, along with IRS management, allocates IRS's appropriation to IRS teams doing the implementation work. By involving the CFO in reviewing identified risks, the risk plan ensures that the CFO is aware of any risks related to the availability of resources. Regularly scheduled meetings between the CFO and PPACA implementation leadership also serve to facilitate discussion of the risks related to resource allocation. To the extent that IRS provides more specific guidance in the risk plan on verifying resources and updates its cost estimate for PPACA implementation, IRS will enhance its ability to manage risks related to allocating resources in an efficient manner.

Managing Risk in Coordinating with Partner Agencies

IRS and HHS developed an informal process for regular communication on project management, consisting of meetings several times per week to monitor progress on deliverables and solicit needed input on IRS activities that affect other agencies.[13] IRS officials expressed confidence

---

[13] We focused on coordination between IRS and HHS because IRS collaborates with HHS more than any other agency in implementing PPACA. Work includes development of IT systems that share data needed for exchange-related work that IRS described as a major challenge.

that the informal system of coordination worked effectively. The agencies also jointly established more formal guiding principles for their implementation efforts in 2010 to clarify goals and objectives.

Although IRS and HHS regularly coordinated, we did not find a formal system for managing risks threatening the agencies' success in achieving their goals. Without a joint tracking system for risks related to the agencies' coordinated efforts, the agencies may duplicate efforts. They could also focus on tracking implementation deadlines while losing sight of risks that pose obstacles to meeting those deadlines.

Managing Risk in Determining the Need for Deadline Extensions and Transitional Relief

IRS's PPACA implementation teams[14] work with Counsel to develop plans for overcoming obstacles that create the need for deadline extensions and transitional relief. The plans are to be guided by three specific criteria—the timing of legislation with respect to the tax year, burden imposed on taxpayers and intermediaries, and IRS effort required—in determining the need for extensions and relief. As of May 2012, seven provisions were granted extensions and relief in consideration of timing issues and the burden imposed criteria. Counsel participates in the risk management process by briefing implementation teams at the outset of work, participating in regular meetings with IRS leadership for PPACA risk management, soliciting comments on guidance from stakeholders and the general public, and helping to monitor progress. Counsel's involvement in these activities as well as the use of specific criteria should help IRS make decisions on granting extensions and relief as the implementation dates approach for major provisions, such as those related to the exchanges in 2014.

Managing Risk in Addressing Compliance and Burden Challenges

We found consistent evidence IRS had taken steps to identify potential compliance challenges. IRS used its Research, Analysis, and Statistics (RAS) organization to help project the volume of tax returns that would be subject to PPACA and help identify the likely population requiring outreach and education. When historical data for similar provisions were available, IRS attempted to use the data to construct a baseline of anticipated results. Counsel solicited formal comments from stakeholders and taxpayers in response to preliminary guidance. IRS made limited use of other means, such as focus groups, to gain insight into compliance and

---

[14] This process involves other offices within the U.S. Department of the Treasury, such as the Office of Tax Policy.

burden challenges facing the public. IRS officials said that they received informal feedback from conversations with other tax stakeholders, such as groups representing taxpayers, tax software developers, and tax preparers. We also saw evidence, such as with tax credits for small employers offering health insurance, that IRS enforcement staff attempted to account for known or suspected compliance risks.[15] The risk plan calls for early warning thresholds that indicate that results are below expectations and we saw evidence that such thresholds are used regularly.

Conclusions

Since our 2011 report, IRS has gained a better understanding of the work and challenges it faces in implementing PPACA. IRS has made varying degrees of progress in implementing our recommendations from 2011. As IRS continues to implement them, IRS leadership will enhance its line of sight over its progress and the challenges that remain.

With expected implementation costs approaching $1 billion as IRS gets closer to major milestones in 2014, careful consideration of risks and alternatives for mitigating those risks is crucial in meeting deadlines and making the best use of taxpayer dollars. While IRS developed a risk management plan for PPACA implementation that meets several leading practices, IRS did not take any actions to implement our 2011 recommendation on assessing mitigation strategies. Further, IRS could take specific steps such as providing additional guidance on how to evaluate potential mitigation strategies and document the rationales for decisions made. Without additional guidance, IRS staff selecting mitigation strategies may not fully evaluate all alternatives or verify that resources are available for the strategy chosen. Not knowing the rationale behind selecting a mitigation strategy over others could hinder future decisions if the original strategy did not work and the original decision makers are no longer involved.

While IRS's PPACA implementation teams generally followed the steps of the risk management plan in identifying and mitigating risks, the plan was not followed when Counsel led pieces of the implementation. If the plan is not followed, risks may not be addressed. Additionally, without a shared

---

[15] GAO, *Small Employer Health Tax Credit: Factors Contributing to Low Use and Complexity*, GAO-12-549 (Washington, D.C.: May 14, 2012).

GAO-12-690 Patient Protection and Affordable Care Act

system for tracking and monitoring risks with partner agencies, such as HHS, the agencies will be more likely to overlook potential challenges or duplicate efforts to mitigate risks.

Recommendations for Executive Action

To strengthen the PPACA risk management plan, we recommend that the Commissioner of Internal Revenue enhance guidance on evaluating risk mitigation alternatives to

- clarify who is responsible for doing the evaluation and making decisions based on the results as well as how they might do the evaluation,
- assure that resources are available for the chosen mitigation strategy, and
- document the mitigation alternatives considered and rationale(s) for the decisions made.

To ensure more consistent implementation of the risk management plan, we recommend that the Commissioner of Internal Revenue take the following two actions:

- ensure that the PPACA risk management plan is applied to provisions in which the Office of Chief Counsel assumes lead responsibility for implementation, and
- develop agreements with HHS (and other external parties as needed) on a system to record and track details on decisions made or to be made to ensure that risks are identified and mitigated.

Agency Comments and Our Evaluation

In a June 1, 2012, letter responding to a draft of this report (which is reprinted in app. IV), the IRS Deputy Commissioner for Services and Enforcement provided comments on our findings and recommendations as well as information on IRS efforts and progress to date on its PPACA implementation.

IRS agreed with our first recommendation to enhance guidance in its PPACA risk management plan related to evaluating risk mitigation alternatives. Specifically, IRS agreed to revise its plan to (1) clarify responsibilities for doing the evaluation and making related decisions, (2) assure that resources are available for the mitigation strategy chosen, and (3) document the alternatives considered and the rationale(s) for decisions made.

IRS also agreed with our two recommendations to ensure more consistent application of its risk management plan. First, IRS agreed to revise its plan to address the use of the plan for provisions being led by the Office of Chief Counsel. Second, IRS agreed to consult with HHS on the best approach to document and track decisions, risks, or both that affect both agencies. In that this recommendation referenced HHS specifically and possibly other external parties in identifying and mitigating these "joint" risks, we encourage IRS to take similar coordinated steps, as needed, when risks arise that affect IRS and these other parties.

We are sending copies of this report to appropriate congressional committees, the Commissioner of Internal Revenue, the Secretary of the Treasury, the Chairman of the IRS Oversight Board, and the Director of the Office of Management and Budget. In addition, the report is available at no charge on the GAO website at http://www.gao.gov.

If you or your staffs have any questions or wish to discuss the material in this report further, please contact me at (202) 512-9110 or at whitej@gao.gov. Contact points for our Offices of Congressional Relations and Public Affairs may be found on the last page of this report. GAO staff who made key contributions to this report are listed in appendix V.

James R. White
Director, Tax Issues
Strategic Issues

Appendix I: Scope and Methodology

To assess IRS's progress in addressing our 2011 recommendations for improving PPACA implementation efforts, we compared IRS's planned and ongoing actions to leading practices described in our report. We analyzed IRS documentation and data, including program goals, project plans, cost estimates, risk management plans, governance plan, and presentations. We interviewed IRS officials and staff at IRS's National Office, including those in the Office of the Chief Financial Officer (CFO); Office of Chief Counsel; and Services & Enforcement (S&E) and Modernization and Information Technology Services (MITS) Program Management Offices (PMO) to clarify our understanding of IRS's progress and plans for implementing our recommendations.

To assess IRS's risk management plan for PPACA, we compared the contents of IRS's Risk Management Plan, governance plan, and high-level action plans to the criteria outlined by GAO's risk management approach. We met with officials from the S&E PMO to confirm our understanding of the policies and procedures included in IRS's risk management process.

To evaluate how consistently IRS applies its risk management plan for PPACA implementation, we analyzed IRS activities across a sample of PPACA provisions to verify that IRS followed the steps included in its risk plan. To assemble our sample, we identified provisions with the greatest likelihood of adverse effects and potential for the most significant financial consequences if risks were not identified and mitigated. We limited the scope of our sample to the 23 provisions with anticipated revenue and expenditure impacts of over $1 billion over the first 10 years of the legislation, as scored by the Joint Committee of Taxation and Congressional Budget Office. We eliminated 14 provisions to arrive at the final sample of 9 provisions based on the following criteria (see app. III for the 9 provisions in the sample).

For example, since we focused on IRS's use of its PPACA risk plan, which was initially drafted in 2011, we removed six provisions, including:

- Four provisions that were implemented prior to the existence of IRS's risk plan:
  - Section 10909 related to an adoption tax credit,
  - Section 1408 (HCERA) related to the exclusion of cellulosic biofuel from a tax credit,
  - Section 9003 related to repealing a tax exclusion in health flexible spending arrangements, and

- Section 9004 related to a tax on distributions from certain health savings accounts.
- Two provisions for which implementation had not started:
  - Section 9005 related to the limits on health flexible spending arrangements, and
  - Section 9001 related to an excise tax on high-cost employer-provided health insurance plans.

To target provisions with the greatest likelihood of adverse effects from a failure to mitigate risks, we removed another seven provisions, including:

- Three provisions because IRS had identified only low level risks for them:
  - Section 9013 related to the medical expense deduction threshold,
  - Section 1405 (HCERA) related to an excise tax on medical devices, and
  - Section 9012 related to the elimination of an employer deduction for a retiree prescription drug subsidy.
- Four provisions for which only 1 risk had been identified:
  - Section 1322 related to a tax exemption for start-up nonprofit health insurers,
  - Section 6301 related to a fee on health insurance plans,
  - Section 10907 related to an excise tax on tanning salon services, and
  - Section 9010 related to an annual fee on health insurers.

Finally, because of overlap in the remaining provisions that required very similar work for IRS, we removed a provision from Section 9015 related to an increase of the Hospital Insurance tax on wages over a specified threshold.

We asked IRS to provide evidence of its risk management activity in four key areas. For three of these areas—resource allocation, coordination with external partners, and compliance and burden challenges—we also sought this documentation as part of our work on the nine provisions. We analyzed IRS's responses and documentation, including risk logs, to determine what gaps, if any, existed between the steps called for by the risk plan and the actions that IRS took. We interviewed IRS officials and staff responsible for PPACA implementation, including officials from the PMOs for S&E and MITS, Office of the Chief Counsel, and Office of the CFO, and officials from the Department of Health and Human Services in conducting this work.

For the risks related to the fourth key area—deadline extensions and other transitional relief—we interviewed officials in the Office of Chief Counsel. We sought information on their approach to understand how Chief Counsel coordinates with implementation teams about risks as decisions are considered and made about the extensions and relief.

We conducted this performance audit from August 2011 to June 2012 in accordance with generally accepted government auditing standards. Those standards require that we plan and perform the audit to obtain sufficient, appropriate evidence to provide a reasonable basis for our findings and conclusions based on our audit objectives. We believe that the evidence obtained provides a reasonable basis for our findings and conclusions based on our audit objectives.

Appendix II: How IRS Fulfills GAO Risk Management Criteria

To assess how IRS's revised risk plan meets the criteria for each of GAO's risk management framework stages, we compared the criteria for each stage of the framework to the steps included in each of the stages of IRS's risk management plan. Table 7 shows how IRS's risk management plan meets the criteria for the risk management framework.

Table 7: How IRS Fulfills GAO Risk Management Criteria

GAO risk management framework stages	IRS risk management plan stages	How IRS fulfills GAO criteria
Strategic Goals, Objectives, and Constraints	N/A	The framework calls for documentation of (a) strategic goals and objectives of the initiative and (b) the steps needed to attain those results. IRS's risk management plan does not explicitly address goals, objectives, and constraints. Instead, those strategic plans and objectives are communicated through IRS's "ACA Governance Plan," which communicates the agency's implementation goals and objectives broadly to implementation teams. Additionally, steps to attaining program goals are contained in the agency's high level action plans (HLAP) for PPACA projects.
Risk Assessment	Identification	The framework calls for documentation of standard operating procedures designed to identify (a) what can go wrong, (b) the likelihood of a risk occurring, and (c) the consequences of an occurrence. In its identification and tracking stages, IRS has established a consistent process for meeting these criteria.
	Tracking	
Alternatives Evaluation	Resolution/Mitigation	The framework calls for a consistent process by which to evaluate potential mitigation strategies using a variety of criteria, particularly cost-benefit analyses. While IRS provides general criteria for teams to evaluate alternatives, including cost, it does not outline specific guidance for performing this analysis.
Management Selection		The framework calls for a consistent process by which IRS (a) selects a risk mitigation strategy; (b) allocates resources to pursue that strategy; and (c) documents decisions, including the rationale behind the decisions. IRS's plan does not address procedures for selecting strategies or allocating resources for selected strategies, nor does it outline protocols for documenting decisions made.
Implementation and Monitoring	Reporting	The framework calls for documentation of processes to (a) monitor progress of mitigation strategies and establish timelines and (b) detect failed strategies in need of revision. IRS meets these criteria through its biweekly meetings with workstream risk managers, BOD executive leads, and PPACA senior leadership. These meetings allow for continued review of risks and escalation of risk ownership as risks develop. IRS plans to develop performance measures by July 1, 2012, to help identify strategies in need of revision.

Source: GAO analysis.

GAO-12-690 Patient Protection and Affordable Care Act

Appendix III: Provisions Evaluated for Consistent Use of Risk Management Plan

In evaluating IRS's responses to a sample of nine PPACA provisions, we found that IRS generally followed the plan to identify, track and report risks. As discussed in our report, exceptions were (1) IRS did not consistently evaluate potential risk mitigation strategies in the Resolution/Mitigation stage of its risk plan, and (2) the risk plan was not used when the Office of Chief Counsel led the implementation of provisions related to a reinsurance program for early retirees and the economic substance doctrine. Table 8 shows the results of our evaluation.

Table 8: Consistency with Which IRS Used Its Risk Plan in Implementing Selected PPACA Provisions

Provision	Description	Identification	Tracking	Resolution/ mitigation	Reporting
Patient Protection and Affordable Care Act (PPACA), Pub. L. No. 111-148, 124 Stat. 119 (Mar. 23, 2010)					
1102[a]	Establishes a temporary reinsurance program to provide reimbursement for a portion of the cost of providing health insurance coverage to early retirees.	○	○	○	○
1401	Provides premium assistance refundable tax credits for applicable taxpayers who purchase insurance through a state exchange, paid directly to the insurance plans monthly or to individuals who pay out-of-pocket at the end of the taxable year.	●	●	◑	●
1402	Provides a cost-sharing subsidy for applicable taxpayers to reduce annual out-of-pocket deductibles.	●	●	◑	●
1421	Provides nonrefundable tax credits for qualified small employers (no more than 25 full-time equivalents (FTE) with annual wages averaging no more than $50,000) for contributions made on behalf of its employees for premiums for qualified health plans.	●	●	◑	●
1501	Requires all U.S. citizens and legal residents and their dependents to maintain minimum essential insurance coverage unless exempted starting in 2014 and imposes a fine on those failing to maintain such coverage.	●	●	◑	●
1513	Imposes a penalty on large employers (50+ FTEs) who (1) do not offer coverage for all of their full-time employees, offer unaffordable minimum essential coverage, or offer plans with high out-of-pocket costs and (2) have at least one full-time employee certified as having purchased health insurance through a state exchange and was eligible for a tax credit or subsidy.	●	●	◑	●

GAO-12-690 Patient Protection and Affordable Care Act

Provision	Description	Identification	Tracking	Resolution/ mitigation	Reporting
9008	Imposes a fee on each covered entity engaged in the business of manufacturing or importing branded prescription drugs.	●	●	◑	●
Health Care and Education Reconciliation Act of 2010 (HCERA), Pub. L. No. 111-152, 124 Stat. 1029 (Mar. 30, 2010)					
1402	Imposes an unearned income Medicare contribution tax of 3.8 percent on individuals, estates, and trusts on the lesser of net investment income or the excess of modified adjusted gross income (AGI + foreign earned income) over a threshold of $200,000 (individual) or $250,000 (joint).	●	●	◑	●
1409[b]	Clarifies and enhances the applications of the economic substance doctrine and imposes penalties for underpayments attributable to transaction lacking economic substance.	○	○	○	○

Legend:

●   Consistently followed risk management plan while addressing risks related to implementation

◑   Partially followed risk management plan while addressing risks related to implementation

○   Did not consistently follow risk management plan while addressing risks related to implementation

Source: GAO analysis based on IRS data.

[a]Implementation of this provision was led by the Office of Chief Counsel. The ACA Risk Management Plan was not used to track risks related to the implementation of this provision.

[b]Implementation of this provision was led by the Office of Chief Counsel. The ACA Risk Management Plan was not used to track risks related to the implementation of this provision.

Appendix IV: Comments from the Internal Revenue Service

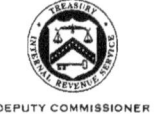

DEPARTMENT OF THE TREASURY
INTERNAL REVENUE SERVICE
WASHINGTON, D.C. 20224

DEPUTY COMMISSIONER

June 1, 2012

Mr. James R. White
Director, Tax Issues
Strategic Issues Team
United States Government Accountability Office
Washington, DC 20548

Dear Mr. White:

Thank you for the opportunity to review your draft report entitled "PATIENT PROTECTION AND AFFORDABLE CARE ACT: IRS Managing Implementation Risks But Its Approach Could Be Refined" (GAO-12-690, Job Code 450943). As you noted, IRS's implementation of the Affordable Care Act (ACA) is a significant undertaking and we are pleased your report acknowledges the progress we have made thus far. We have implemented many of the tax provisions contained in the ACA but more work remains to be done. We appreciate the input you have provided as we continue our implementation efforts.

We agree with your recommendations to refine and improve our risk management process. The enclosed response addresses each of your recommendations.

Sincerely,

Steven T. Miller
Deputy Commissioner for Services and Enforcement

Enclosure

Enclosure

GAO Recommendations and IRS Responses to GAO Draft Report
PATIENT PROTECTION AND AFFORDABLE CARE ACT
IRS Managing Implementation Risks But Its Approach Could Be Refined
GAO-12-690

Recommendation: To strengthen the PPACA risk management plan, we recommend that the Commissioner of Internal Revenue enhance guidance on evaluating risk mitigation alternatives to:
- Clarify who is responsible for doing the evaluation and making decisions based on the results as well as how they might do the evaluation.
- Assure that resources are available for the chosen mitigation strategy.
- Document the mitigation alternatives considered and rationale(s) for the decisions made.

Comments: We agree with this recommendation. We will revise our risk management plan to address these issues.

Recommendation: To ensure more consistent implementation of the risk management plan, we recommend that the Commissioner of Internal Revenue ensure that the PPACA risk management plan is applied to provisions in which the Office of Chief Counsel assumes lead responsibility for implementation.

Comments: We agree with this recommendation. We will revise our risk management plan to address the application of the plan to provisions assigned to Chief Counsel.

Recommendation: To ensure more consistent implementation of the risk management plan, we recommend that the Commissioner of Internal Revenue develop agreements with HHS (and other external parties as needed) on a system to record and track details on decisions made or to be made to ensure that risks are identified and mitigated.

Comments: We agree with this recommendation. We will consult with HHS and determine the best approach to document and track decisions and/or risks which impact us both.

Appendix V: GAO Contact and Staff Acknowledgments

GAO Contact	James R. White, (202) 512-9110, whitej@gao.gov
Staff Acknowledgments	In addition to the to the individual named above, Thomas Short, Assistant Director; Ben Atwater; Linda Baker; Amy Bowser; Dean Campbell; Jennifer Echard; Rebecca Gambler; Meredith Graves; Sairah Ijaz; Sherrice Kerns; Donna Miller; Patrick Murray; Sabine Paul; and Cynthia Saunders made key contributions to this report.

Related GAO Products

IRS 2013 Budget: Continuing to Improve Information on Program Costs and Results Could Aid in Resource Decision Making. GAO-12-603. Washington, D.C.: June 8, 2012.

Small Employer Health Tax Credit: Factors Contributing to Low Use and Complexity. GAO-12-549. Washington, D.C.: May 14, 2012.

Patient Protection and Affordable Care Act: IRS Should Expand Its Strategic Approach to Implementation. GAO-11-719. Washington, D.C.: June 25, 2011.

GAO Cost Estimating and Assessment Guide: Best Practices for Developing and Managing Capital Program Costs. GAO-09-3SP. Washington, D.C.: March 2, 2009.

Risk Management: Further Refinements Needed to Assess Risks and Prioritize Protective Measures at Ports and Other Critical Infrastructure. GAO-06-91. Washington, D.C.: December 15, 2005.

(450943)